Salvador Jiménez Mejines
Felipe Arteaga García
Jorge Ibarra Aguilar

Therapeutic alliance in pediatric patients with status epilepticus

Salvador Jiménez Mejines
Felipe Arteaga García
Jorge Ibarra Aguilar

Therapeutic alliance in pediatric patients with status epilepticus

Hospital del Niño DIF, Hidalgo

ScienciaScripts

Imprint

Any brand names and product names mentioned in this book are subject to trademark, brand or patent protection and are trademarks or registered trademarks of their respective holders. The use of brand names, product names, common names, trade names, product descriptions etc. even without a particular marking in this work is in no way to be construed to mean that such names may be regarded as unrestricted in respect of trademark and brand protection legislation and could thus be used by anyone.

Cover image: www.ingimage.com

This book is a translation from the original published under ISBN 978-620-2-11684-8.

Publisher:
Sciencia Scripts
is a trademark of
Dodo Books Indian Ocean Ltd. and OmniScriptum S.R.L publishing group

120 High Road, East Finchley, London, N2 9ED, United Kingdom
Str. Armeneasca 28/1, office 1, Chisinau MD-2012, Republic of Moldova, Europe
Printed at: see last page
ISBN: 978-620-5-74636-3

Presentation

The present book allows us to talk about the cases presented on Epilepsy, which is a generalised epileptic seizure in children and adults, one that lasts five minutes or more, or two or more seizures without recovery of alertness in a period of 30 minutes.

Status epilepticus is the most common paediatric neurological emergency, with an incidence of 18-23 per 100,000 children per year. This condition has a significant morbidity and mortality when not treated appropriately.

The research focused on evaluating the therapeutic alliance of paediatricians to the treatment algorithm for paediatric patients with status epilepticus at the Hospital del Niño DIF Hidalgo.

For this purpose, a quantitative, observational and prospective study was carried out to describe the therapeutic alliance of doctors to the treatment algorithm for paediatric patients in status epilepticus at the Hospital del Niño DIF Hidalgo.

As general information in the Hospital del Niño DIF Hidalgo, 24 patients have been registered from December 2020 to December 2021 (13 female cases (54.1%) and 11 males (45.9%), with an average of 2 patients per month. With an average age of 36 months. These were classified as imminent status epilepticus, 19 cases (77.9%), 4 established (16.4%), 3 refractory (5.7%) and there were no supe refractory cases.

Adherence to the treatment algorithm for patients with status epilepticus was 58.33%. Adequate therapeutic adherence to the treatment algorithm for paediatric patients reduces the time to remission of status epilepticus, thereby reducing morbidity and mortality in these patients.

Table of Contents

Glossary of terms

Epileptic seizure: A clinical manifestation, whether motor, sensory, sensory, psychic or other, secondary to an abnormal, synchronised and excessive discharge of cortical neurons; these are usually abrupt, brief, paroxysmal and self-limited episodes.

Epilepsy: A disorder of the central nervous system (CNS) characterised by the recurrence of two or more epileptic seizures in the absence of an identifiable acute immediate cause.

Epileptic syndrome: A set of signs and symptoms that define a particular type of epilepsy. A set of entities grouping patients with common clinical, electroencephalographic, aetiological, pathophysiological and prognostic features.

Status Epilepticus: The International League Against Epilepsy defines a generalised epileptic seizure in children and adults as a seizure lasting five minutes or more, or two or more seizures without recovery of alertness within 30 minutes.

Impending status epilepticus: A seizure lasting less than 5 minutes.

Established status epilepticus: status epilepticus lasting more than 5 minutes and less than 30 minutes.

Refractory status epilepticus: unresponsive to first- and second-line treatment; lasts 60-120 minutes.

Supra-refractory status epilepticus: if after 24 hours of anaesthetics the EE continues or recurs.

List of tables, graphs and illustrations.

Pictures
- Table 1: Algorithm of the patient in status epilepticus at the Hospital del Niño DIF, Hidalgo. Page 12.
- Table 2: Classification of status epilepticus ILAE 2017 Page 17.
- Table 3: Classification of status epilepticus by semiology ILAE 2017 Page 21.
- Table 4: Classification of status epilepticus by aetiology ILAE 2017 Page 22.
- Table 5: Classification of status epilepticus by EEG ILAE 2017 Page 22.
- Table 6: Classification of status epilepticus by age ILAE 2017 Page 22.
- Table 7: Comparative table of results on Status epilepticus 2021 vs. 2016 Page 22.

Graphics
- Figure 1: Sex of patients Page 40
- Graph 2: Age of patients Page 40
- Figure 3: Classification of Status Epilepticus Page 41
- Figure 4: Therapeutic alliance of physicians to the treatment algorithm for patients with status epilepticus at the Hospital del Niño DIF, Hidalgo. Page 41.

1. Introduction

The International League Against Epilepsy (ILAE) defines Status Epilepticus (SE) as a condition resulting from the failure of the mechanism responsible for terminating the seizure or the restarting mechanism, leading to an abnormally long seizure. It is a condition in which there may be long-term consequences including: (3)

1. Neuronal death.
2. Neuronal injury.
3. Alterations in the neural network.

Stages of status epilepticus:
1. Five minutes: EE imminent, time to initiate therapeutic measures.
2. Thirty minutes: EE established.
3. Refractory EE: does not respond to first- and second-line treatment; lasts 60-120 minutes.
4. Supra-refractory EE: if after 24 hours of anaesthetics the EE continues or recurs (5).

Status epilepticus is the most common paediatric neurological emergency, with an incidence of 18-23 per 100,000 children per year. This condition has a significant morbidity and mortality when not treated appropriately. It is associated with a short-term mortality of 0-3% and a long-term mortality of 7% (1). Seizure EE can be focal in 29% of cases or generalised in 36% and accounts for 90% of cases in children, with refractory seizures in 30% of all cases (2). Generalised seizures occur in 35% of focal seizures. Most children under five years of age will typically have generalised tonic-clonic seizures (GTCS) lasting less than five minutes (8).

Status epilepticus can be classified based on four main axes, which may not always be determined: semiology, aetiology, electroencephalography correlation and age (4).

- Axis 1 (semiology). Two criteria are considered: the presence or absence of motor symptoms and signs and the degree (qualitative or quantitative) of altered consciousness.

- Axis 2 (aetiology). It is sometimes difficult to determine the cause of SE, so two groups are suggested, known or unknown cause.

- Axis 3 (electroencephalography correlation). In most first or second level hospital centres, electroencephalography (EEG) equipment is not always available; if it can be performed, it is suggested that it be done immediately and, based on descriptive series and consensus, we can describe six electrical patterns.

- Axis 4 (age). Important axis, because the clinical manifestations of SE can vary (4).

The most common triggers for seizures include emotional stress or anxiety, sleep deprivation, missed doses of medication (non-adherence to treatment), menstruation and alcohol consumption. Less common triggers include olfactory, tactile or auditory stimuli, dehydration, contact with hot water and fasting (11).

Two-thirds of patients respond to the first treatment, and if timely and appropriate action is taken, the prognosis for these patients is generally good. With proper drug selection and individualised diagnostic approach, seizure control can be achieved, and the patient should be managed and monitored, as with any individual suffering from epilepsy (6).

Unfortunately, between 3 and 33% die from status epilepticus itself or from complications caused by status epilepticus. A management algorithm during status epilepticus improves prognosis and optimises resources (13).

Several prognostic factors are important in predicting the outcome of EE: precipitating cause, age, seizure duration and response to treatment. The highest mortality groups are patients with anoxia or underlying pathologies and, to a lesser extent, those with epilepsy and low concentrations of antiepileptic drugs. Immediate control of EE and timely detection of the cause are essential, as they have a direct impact on morbidity and mortality (15).

The neurological sequelae can be very diverse; however, those of the cognitive sphere predominate, because these patients are subjected to diffuse cerebral hypoxia by various mechanisms, so that we can also find motor and sensory sequelae (17).

The Hospital del Niño DIF Hidalgo reported a prevalence of EE of 19 cases per 1000 inhabitants in 2016 in the paediatric age group (from birth to 16 years). The recorded mortality was 22.7%, the first cause was cerebral ischaemia 60% and the second cause was septic shock in 30% (19).

Based on national and international guidelines on Status Epilepticus, an algorithm for the treatment of patients with status epilepticus was created at the Hospital del Niño DIF, Hidalgo, which since 2016 has been established as a guideline to follow in the choice of effective treatment and dosage, in accordance with the recommendations established by the American Epilepsy Society and the organisational context with the aim of reducing morbidity and mortality in patients with EE who are treated at the Hospital Niño DIF de Hidalgo (7).

According to the findings of this research, the advantages of using the algorithm are as follows:

- Any patient admitted to the emergency department with status epilepticus as an established status epilepticus should receive first- and second-line direct management without delay, respecting the dose, route and infusion indications of each of the drugs, as established in the algorithm.

- A permanent stock of phenytoin, valproic acid and levetiracetam should be kept in the emergency department.

- The main triggering aetiology of status epilepticus in the Niño DIF Hospital was infectious, so this pathology should be addressed, ruled out and treated (7).

The algorithm consists of 4 phases:

1. Stabilisation phase (0-5 minutes) with monitoring, vital signs management and laboratory tests.

2. First-line treatment phase (5-20 minutes) with administration of benzodiazepines.

3. Second-line therapy phase (20-40 minutes) with administration of an antiepileptic drug other than benzodiazepines when the first line has failed.

4. Third-line therapy phase (40-60 minutes), during which the administration of another second-line drug or a different general anaesthetic drug is indicated (7).

Table 1: Algorithm of the patient in status epilepticus at the Hospital del Niño DIF, Hidalgo.

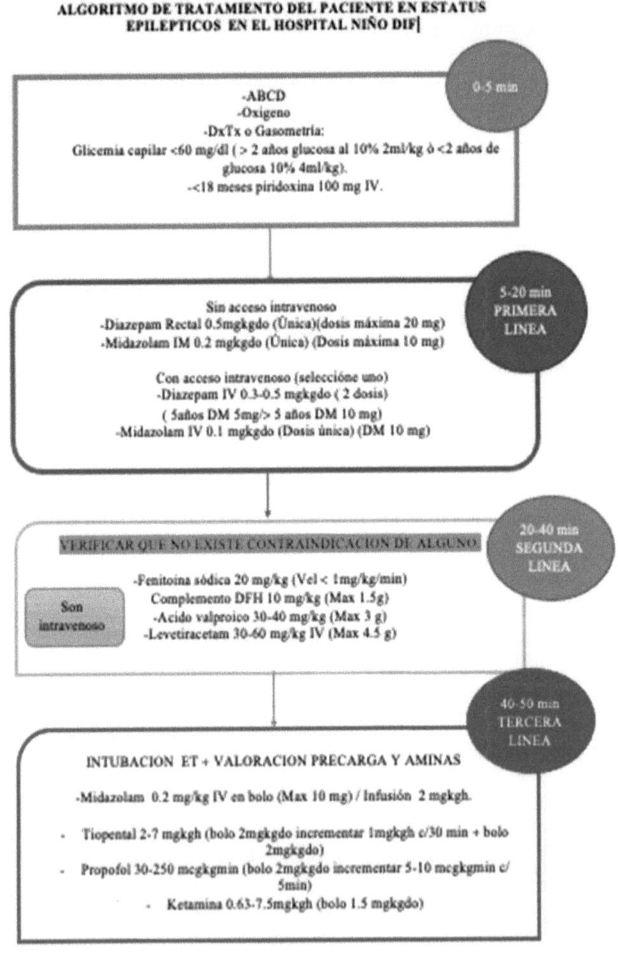

Source: Algoritmo de tratamiento del Paciente en Estado Epiléptico en el Hospital de Niño DIF Hidalgo.

At present, this algorithm has not been applied, so there is a need to carry out a study on physician adherence in order to determine its effectiveness and to be able to improve it or establish it as the best option for the treatment of patients with status epilepticus who are admitted to the Emergency Department of the Niño DIF Hospital.

2. Problem statement

The International League Against Epilepsy proposes the operational definition of status epilepticus (SE) as a generalised tonic-clonic seizure in children and adults, lasting five minutes or more, or two or more seizures without recovery of alertness within 30 minutes (4).

Epilepsy is one of the diseases that most affects patients' quality of life due to its neurobiological, psychological and social implications. Epileptic seizures (SEs) are a common cause of admission to the Emergency Department (ED) and account for 1 million or 1% of all ED visits (20).

The disease currently affects nearly 70 million people worldwide. The prevalence of epilepsy in low- and middle-income countries (LMIC) is about twice as high as in high-income countries. In Mexico, epilepsy has a prevalence of 10.8-20 cases per 1,000 population, or 1.08-2% of the total population (13).

Clinical practice guidelines state that 8-10% of the population is at risk of having a seizure and a 3% chance of developing epilepsy, non-epileptic events are twice as frequent as epilepsy and the diagnosis is uncertain in 20% of cases at the time of the first seizure (15).

Current research has established that poor pre-hospital management or delayed initiation of treatment of EE increases morbidity and mortality in these patients (9).

Studies report that in patients with adequate therapy, mortality can be as low as 8%, while it can be as high as 45% in those with insufficient therapy. Therapeutic alliance to a treatment protocol was associated with better seizure control and shorter hospital and intensive care stay (11).

However, in our country there is not yet an ideal standard protocol for the treatment of patients with ES; there are multiple clinical guidelines and protocols based on clinical practice, consensus opinions and the availability of drugs at the local level. At the Hospital del Niño DIF Hidalgo, an algorithm for the treatment of patients with EE was created in 2016, with the aim of reducing morbidity and mortality in patients with EE, which has not yet been fully and correctly implemented to date, which is why the research question arises: (7).

2.1 Research question

What is the therapeutic alliance of physicians to the treatment algorithm for paediatric patients with status epilepticus at the Hospital del Niño DIF Hidalgo?

3. Justification

Worldwide, the annual incidence of EE in children is estimated to be between 17-23 cases per 100,000 children, of which 10-40% develop refractory EE, with a mortality of 16-42.5%. When the duration of EE is longer than 2 hours, neurological sequelae and cognitive disorders increase, reaching an incidence of up to 48% (1).

Epilepsy is most common in the paediatric age group, and the male sex is the most affected· In Mexico, 400 to 800 new cases per 100 000 children are reported each year· The substrate for the genesis of epilepsy can be genetic and acquired· Genetic abnormalities contribute to the development of acquired epilepsy by increasing a person's predisposition to trigger seizures by environmental factors (5).

In the Hospital del Niño DIF Hidalgo, in 2016 a treatment algorithm was developed based on international and national research and treatment guidelines, however, it has not been fully implemented, so the need arises to know the results that this will have after its application in this institution, to determine whether or not there is a positive impact on patient care, so the results of this research will allow decisions to be made to provide timely care or the redesign of the algorithm to correctly treat this pathology.

4. Objectives

4.1 General Objective

To evaluate the therapeutic alliance of physicians to the treatment algorithm for paediatric patients with status epilepticus at the Hospital del Niño DIF Hidalgo.

4.2 Specific Objectives

1. Determine the number of patients who were treated with the treatment algorithm for patients with status epilepticus at the Hospital del Niño DIF Hidalgo.

2. To identify the time in which status epilepticus is successfully jugulated and the average length of in-hospital stay of patients.

3. To describe the therapeutic alliance to the algorithm according to the times, doses, route and infusion of the drugs of choice in the first, second and third line treatments according to the algorithm of treatment of the patient in status epilepticus in the Hospital Niño DIF Hidalgo.

5. Hypothesis

H1.
Treating physicians adhere properly and correctly to the treatment algorithm for paediatric patients with status epilepticus at the Hospital del Niño DIF Hidalgo.

H0.
Treating physicians do not adequately and correctly adhere to the treatment algorithm for paediatric patients with status epilepticus at the Hospital del Niño DIF Hidalgo.

6. Theoretical Framework

A seizure is the transient occurrence of signs and/or symptoms caused by excessive abnormal neuronal activity in the brain.

A diagnosis of epilepsy is established in any of the following situations:

- Two or more unprovoked or reflexive seizures occurring more than 24 hours apart.

- An unprovoked or reflex crisis and a probability of future crises of at least 60% (similar range to the general recurrence risk after two unprovoked crises occurring in the next 10 years).

- The diagnosis of an epileptic syndrome (4).

The ILAE decided to modify the 1981 seizure classification system and update the 2010 classification· The classification has three sections depending on the patient's onset symptoms: seizures of focal onset, seizures of generalised onset and seizures of unknown onset. Focal onset seizures originate within networks limited to one hemisphere, they can be localised or more widely distributed. Generalised seizures are those that originate at one point with a broad and rapid involvement of bilaterally distributed networks. And crises where it cannot be decided whether they are focal or generalised in onset with an 80% confidence level, should be considered to be of unknown onset (3).

Table 2: ILAE 2017 seizure classification

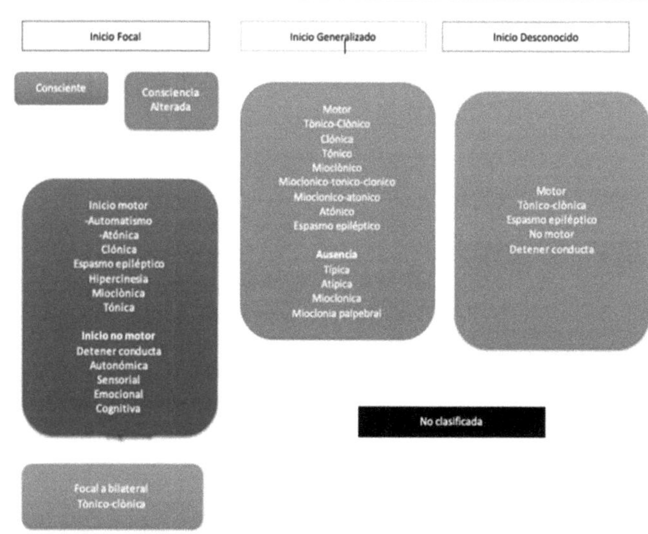

Source: International League Against Epilepsy 2017.

Signs and symptoms of focal seizures:

- Motor. Involvement of the musculature in any form, an increase (positive) or decrease (negative) in muscle contraction to produce a movement. The most common are: motor arrest, asthmatic, clonic, dysarthria, dystonic, pelvic thrust, hypokinetic, hyperkinetic, incoordination, Jacksonian, myoclonic, paralysis, paresis, pedalling, fencer's stance and versive (12).

- The most common clinical confusion is to differentiate between clonic and myoclonic seizures. A clonic seizure is a movement, either symmetrical or asymmetrical, that is repetitive, regular and involves the same muscle groups. Myoclonic seizure is a sudden, brief (< 100 ms), involuntary, single or multiple contraction of muscles or muscle groups of variable topography (axial, proximal limb, distal). Myoclonus is less repetitive and sustained (12).

- Automatisms. More or less coordinated motor activity that usually occurs when cognition is impaired and in which the subject is then usually (but not always) amnesic. Usually resembling a voluntary movement, the most frequent are:

aggression, manual, facial gold, perseverative, sexual, undressing, vocalisation, walking or running (2).

- Sensory. Related to sensations, therefore, they are not signs in this case, but only symptoms. The most frequently reported are: auditory, gustatory, olfactory, somatosensory, vestibular, visual and pain specifically (14).

- Emotional. These are crises that present as an emotion as an initial prominent feature, such as fear, spontaneous joy or euphoria, laughter, crying, occurring in bursts or outbursts (18).

- Cognitive. The most frequently reported data in this group are: acalculia, aphasia, attention disturbance, phenomena of what has already been seen or never seen, dysphasia, delusions, memory disturbance, forced thinking, altered response or hallucination (12).

- Autonomic. Impaired function of the autonomic nervous system, which may involve cardiovascular, pupillary, diaphoresis, gastrointestinal, vasomotor and thermoregulatory functions (13).

Generalised epileptic seizures.

They are divided into crises with motor or non-motor symptoms.
Motor symptoms include generalised tonic-clonic seizures, clonic, tonic, myoclonic, myoclonic-tonic-clonic, myoclonus-clonic, atonic and epileptic spasm, and non-motor symptoms include absence seizures. A myoclonic-tonic-clonic seizure is a type of generalised seizure that was not included in previous classifications. These seizures involve one or more bilateral (myoclonic) jerks of the limbs, followed by a tonic-clonic seizure. Atonic is a seizure with sudden loss or decrease of muscle tone involving the musculature of the head, trunk, jaw or limbs (9).

The epileptic spasm is usually more sustained than a myoclonic movement, but not as sustained as a tonic seizure, which often occurs in clusters or bouts. Infantile spasms are the most common, but can occur at all ages (18).

Absence seizures are described in four possible forms of presentation: typical absences, atypical absences, myoclonic absences and absences with palpebral myoclonus (15).

The typical absence is of sudden onset, interrupting ongoing activity, fixed gaze, the patient does not respond when spoken to, lasting from seconds to half a minute and with very rapid recovery. It is important to remember that the word absence is not synonymous with gaze fixation, as this can also be found in focal onset seizures (12).

Atypical absence is an absence seizure with changes in tone that are more pronounced than in typical absence, the onset or termination is not abrupt. In myoclonic absence, there is a sudden, brief (< 100 ms), involuntary, non-repetitive, non-sustained twitching and absence. In absence with palpebral myoclonus, eyelid twitching is observed at a frequency of less than 3 per second, commonly with upwardly deviated eyes, usually lasting less than 10 seconds, often precipitated by eye closure, with a high possibility of photosensitivity (2).

Status epilepticus:

The International League Against Epilepsy proposes the operational definition of status epilepticus (SE) as a generalised epileptic seizure in children and adults, lasting five minutes or more, or two or more seizures without recovery of alertness within 30 minutes (this includes most generalised epileptic seizures). It is a condition resulting from the failure to initiate inhibitory mechanisms responsible for the termination of a seizure and the persistence of mechanisms that favour the prolongation of a seizure (4).

A generalised motor SE is one with five or more minutes of generalised motor activity or recurrent critical activity without returning to a baseline state. It accounts for 45-75% of all SEs (3).

For focal SE with altered consciousness there is insufficient scientific information, however, it is suggested to define it as an epileptic seizure lasting 10 minutes or two or more seizures without recovery of alertness within 60 minutes. For absence SE, there is no scientific evidence to define the times, but it is proposed to define it as an absence seizure lasting 10 to 15 minutes or more (18).

It can be classified based on four main axes, which may not always be determined: semiology, aetiology, electroencephalographic correlation and age (4).

<table>
<tr><td>

A. With prominent motor symptoms
A1. SE convulsive:
   - A1a. Generalised convulsive
   - A1b. Focal evolving to bilateral convulsive.
   - A1c. It is not known whether it started focal or generalised
A2. Myoclonic SE (prominent myoclonic jerks)
   - A2a. without comma
   - A2b. With comma
A3. Motor focus:
   - A3a. Jacksoniana
   - A3b. EPC
   - A3c. Adversive
   - A3d. Oculoclonic
   - A3e. Ictal paresis or focal inhibitory seizures
 A4. Tonic status
A5. Hyperkinetic SE
B. Non-Prominent Motor Symptoms (NMSP)
B1. EENC with coma (including subtle SE) (note: excludes prominent myoclonus).
 B2. EENC without comma:
   - B2a. Generalised: typical absence, atypical absence and myoclonic status-absence
   - B2b. Focal (non-motor):
   -No compromise of consciousness: different types of continuous auras
   -Aphasic status
   -With compromised consciousness (complex partial or dyscognitive)
   - B2c. Unknown if focal or generalised

</td></tr>
</table>

Axis 1 (semiology). Two criteria are considered: the presence or absence of motor symptoms and signs and the degree (qualitative or quantitative) of altered consciousness (4).

Table 3: Classification of epileptic EE by Semiology, ILAE 2017.

Source: International League Against Epilepsy 2017

Axis 2 (aetiology). It is sometimes difficult to determine the cause of SE, so two groups are suggested, known or unknown cause (4):

Cuadro 4: Clasificación del EE epiléptico por etiología, ILAE 2017.

Known cause (symptomatic)
1.- Acute
2.-Remote
3.-Progressive
4.-SE in defined electrical syndromes.

 Of unknown cause (cryptogenic)

Source: International League Against Epilepsy 2017

Axis 3 (electroencephalographic correlation). In most first or second level hospital centres, electroencephalography (EEG) equipment is not always available; if it can be performed, it is suggested that it be done immediately and, based on descriptive series and consensus, we can describe six electrical patterns (4).

Table 5: Classification of epileptic EE by EEG, ILAE 2017.

Description of EEG findings:
- **Localisation:** generalised or bilateral synchronous lateralised, bilateral independent or multifocal
- **Pattern:** periodic discharges, delta rhythmic activity, spike-wave, sharp-wave-slow-wave, etc.
- **Morphology:** number of phases (e.g. three-phase), grapheme sharpness, amplitude, polarity, etc.
- **Time-related characteristics:** prevalence, frequency, duration, daily pattern, stroke rate or percentage, form of onset (abrupt, evolutionary, fluctuating).
- **Modulation:** stimulus-induced or spontaneous
- Effect of intervention (medication) on offloading

Source: International League Against Epilepsy 2017

Axis 4 (age). Important axis, because the clinical manifestations of SE may vary.

Table 6: Classification of epileptic EE by age, ILAE 2017.

<table>
<tr><td>Age:

• Neonatal: 0-30 days
• Infant: 1 month-2 years
• Childhood: 2-12 years
• Adolescence and adulthood: 12-59 years.
• Senile: Over 60 years of age.</td></tr>
</table>

Source: International League Against Epilepsy 2017

Pathophysiology

Epileptic activity is defined as an abnormal, hypersynchronous and anarchic electrical discharge of a group of neurons, which, once initiated, is self-limiting by mechanisms that are not fully elucidated (13).

From experimental models of epileptogenesis, some of the mechanisms involved have been demonstrated; the most prominent and best known are:

a) Alterations in the cellular ionic environment, such as loss of mainly extra- and intracellular $Ca+$ and $K+$ concentrations and balance, respectively, as well as $Na+$, resulting in altered neuronal membrane permeability (19).

b) On the one hand, exaggerated excitatory activity of neurotransmitters (NT) in relation to increased $Ca+$ -input-dependent secretion of aspartate and glutamate, which act on inotropic and metabotropic receptors, of which N-methyl-D-aspartate is the one most associated with seizures; on the other hand, there is a decrease in the activity and/or concentration of gamma-amino butyric acid (GABA) (14).

c) Structural changes in neurons characterised by loss of dendritic spines and the presence of axonal sprouts. However, in the light of new research, there are other phenomena involved in neuronal epileptic behaviour, such as:

- The involvement of glia. Taking into account its physiological role in water, ionic and neurotransmitter balances of neuronal and glial origin in the neuronal microenvironment.

- Oxidative stress and mitochondrial dysfunction are two events that play an unfavourable role in the propagation and perpetuation of epileptic activity.

- The involvement of blood-brain barrier dysfunction as a promoter and co-permeator of the permeability of pro-inflammatory substances that exacerbate excitatory phenomena (18).

The pathophysiological changes that occur during ET are due to complications in the different organs and systems and depend on the duration of ET, therefore, adequate care is essential to minimise them. They can be divided into two periods: early and late. Early period (0 to 30 minutes) in which the regulatory mechanisms remain intact and late period (after approximately 30 minutes) in which there is a progressive failure of the compensatory mechanisms (3).

Stages of status epilepticus:

1. Five minutes: EE imminent, time to initiate therapeutic measures.
2. Thirty minutes: EE established.
3. Refractory EE: does not respond to first- and second-line treatment; lasts 60-120 minutes.
4. Super-refractory EE: if after 24 hours of anaesthetics the EE continues or recurs.

Neurological injury is also the result of the repeated electrical discharge that occurs as a consequence of the altered balance between excitatory neurotransmitters (glutamate, aspartate, acetylcholine) and inhibitory neurotransmitters (GABA). At the biochemical level, there is an increase in intracellular calcium which triggers a cascade of reactions leading to cell membrane rupture, inhibition of protein synthesis and cell necrosis (4).

The initial neurological damage is similar to that caused by ischaemia; gliosis and atrophy develop in a late phase, making the neurological damage epileptogenic. Certain brain areas such as the hippocampus, basal nuclei, cerebellum and middle layers of the cortex are most affected in EE (11).

It is not known exactly how long it takes for a prolonged epileptic seizure to cause damage; in these more vulnerable areas it is estimated to be 20-60 minutes. In the absence EE, in which inhibitory predominance is presumed, there are no detectable anatomical lesions (at least on macroscopic examination). In a first phase and in response to amine discharge, systemic blood pressure and cardiac output increase, cerebral blood flow increases, so that cerebral metabolic needs are appropriately met. However, it is this process that facilitates the development of cardiac and structural alterations in cardiac function (21).

At the pulmonary level, neurovegetative stimulation promotes bronchoconstriction, increased bronchial secretions and consequently airway obstruction. Ventilatory changes are compounded by possible bronchoaspiration favoured by induction of vomiting and apnoea causing sustained diaphragmatic contraction. The end result is hypoxaemia and respiratory acidosis (27).

Sustained muscle contraction can lead to rhabdomyolysis, myoglobinemia, myoglobinuria leading to renal failure due to acute tubular necrosis; this process can also be caused by antiepileptic drugs used in the management of EE. In addition, this process can trigger hyperkalaemia, which favours the development of arrhythmias (33).

As a result of muscle exhaustion, CO_2, lactic acid and metabolic acidosis are generated. Other disturbances that occur as a consequence of hypothalamic dysfunction and sustained muscle contraction are related to the presence of severe hyperthermia, up to 40 °C (22).

It should therefore be borne in mind that hyperthermia in association with other findings such as leukocytosis and pleocytosis with proteinuria in the CSF, which are favoured by sympathetic stimulation, may erroneously induce an infectious aetiology in cases of EE (16).

At the biochemical level, hyperglycaemia induced by sympathetic stimulation will promote insulin release causing hypoglycaemia in those patients with low glycogen stores, in which case this event may lead to worsening of EE and neuronal damage (13).

Finally, as a consequence of peripheral vasodilatation favoured by metabolic acidosis, dehydration caused by hyperthermia and amine depletion, circulatory collapse may occur. Ultimately, EE can lead to multi-organ failure, including liver failure and disseminated intravascular coagulation, and these phenomena can increase the resulting neurological damage (22).

Aetiology

Febrile EE accounts for 5% of all febrile seizures, and is the underlying aetiology in a quarter of all EE episodes in the paediatric age group. Febrile EE accounts for more than two-thirds of EE in children aged 1-2 years. Infection of the central nervous system can be a cause of EE such as meningoencephalitis or encephalitis, either bacterial or viral. Parasitic CNS infections such as neurocysticercosis must also be considered (19).

Among children with pre-existing epilepsy, non-compliance with medication is a frequent cause of EE. In children with epilepsy taking antiepileptic drugs, serum levels should be considered (24).

Electrolyte abnormalities such as hyponatraemia or metabolic abnormalities such as hyperglycaemia or hypoglycaemia may play a role in paediatric EE. Hypocalcaemia may present as EE in neonates. Electrolyte or glucose disturbances have been reported in 6% of children with EE. EE induced by electrolyte abnormalities may be refractory to treatment until the underlying metabolic disturbance is corrected. Blood glucose and electrolytes should be obtained in all children with EE (5).

Toxic ingestion may be suggested by history and should also be considered in cases with unknown aetiology. Toxic ingestion is documented in 3.6% of cases of EE. Serum and urine toxicology may be helpful in establishing a diagnosis in these cases (8).

Seizures and EE may be the initial symptom of traumatic brain injury. Although the clinical history or examination may suggest trauma, in some cases, the history may be unclear (26).

In particular, in cases of non-accidental trauma, the initial history may be incomplete. Non-accidental injury in infants is strongly associated with prolonged seizure activity. In cases where a clear aetiology of EE cannot be identified, neuroimaging should be obtained once the child is stabilised and seizures are controlled (23).

Vascular lesions, such as arterial ischaemic stroke or central venous sinus thrombosis, may present as seizures or EE. A persistent focal neurological finding carries a high suspicion of stroke, although prolonged seizure with a subsequent Todd's palsy may mimic stroke. Patients with focal neurological findings require neuroimaging as part of their evaluation (28).

 Brain computed tomography (CT) can be useful in identifying acute ischaemic stroke and intracranial haemorrhage, although subtle or hyperacute ischaemic lesions may require repeated imaging to identify. Magnetic resonance imaging (MRI) should be considered as part of a patient's evaluation for ES once the patient is sufficiently stable, particularly if there is suspicion of stroke or structural injury not identified on CT (21).

Remote symptomatic causes, such as previous occult CNS injury, cortical dysplasia or vascular malformations (in the absence of acute haemorrhage), may also present as EE. Identification of these causes may require MRI imaging or further laboratory evaluation. Similarly, other acute symptomatic aetiologies, such as CNS autoimmune conditions, may require serological or immunological testing to identify them (17).

Some epilepsy syndromes, such as Dravet syndrome (DS) or severe myoclonic epilepsy of infancy, show a specifically increased risk of developing EE. It is an epileptic encephalopathy characterised by the presence of predominantly fever-triggered seizures during the first year of life in a normally developing infant, followed by epilepsy with different seizure types from the second year onwards. The evolution is towards drug-resistant epilepsy and a stagnation in psychomotor development from the second year of life onwards, leading eventually to moderate to severe cognitive deficit. Mutations in the SCN1A gene have been found in the vast majority of patients (22).

Benign seizure with mild gastroenteritis (BGEC) is an afebrile seizure associated with viral gastroenteritis in a healthy child without fever, dehydration, electrolyte imbalance, meningitis or encephalitis. GCL is most common in children aged 1 to 2 years. Rotavirus is the most common agent of gastroenteritis associated with seizure. They appear between the second and third day of evolution of the infectious process (although they can occur from the previous day up to seven days later) (11).

Seizures are generalised tonic-clonic, sometimes focal, of short duration and very often recur and cluster in the following hours. They do not usually recur after 48 hours. They do not require complementary examinations. Even if they recur, they do not require anticonvulsant treatment. It is only necessary if the seizures are prolonged (90% of cases last less than 5 minutes) (13).

Electroencephalography

Its use in the context of a SE is mandatory and should ideally be continuous and prolonged for at least 24 hours after complete control of the seizure. In the case of generalised convulsive EE, its main contribution is to rule out the persistence of a non-convulsive EE after clinical seizure control has been achieved. In non-convulsive EE, on the other hand, the diagnosis can only be based on this examination. Either subintrusive seizures or continuous, quasi-periodic, or lateralised periodic patterns may be found (20).

Sometimes there may be doubts of interpretation, mainly because of the practical approach to be followed and the need or not for aggressive therapeutic behaviour. Thus, for example, after severe anoxic encephalopathy, the appearance of a periodic pattern with generalised discharges, which may formally be termed non-convulsive EE, represents a very ominous prognosis (33).

In cases of metabolic encephalopathies that generate patterns specifically related to these conditions (three-phase waves), correlation with the clinic is indispensable, as it is not possible to differentiate it from a non-convulsive EE; in this case, the absence of a metabolic encephalopathy and the presence of a clear change of consciousness, especially if it was of abrupt onset, will point to an EE (17).

Treatment

The initial treatment strategy includes simultaneous assessment and management of the airway (secure it with advanced management if necessary), ventilation and circulation (obtain intravenous access), administration of abortive treatment, determination of the underlying cause and detection of life-threatening aetiologies such as meningitis or intracranial lesions (4).

All patients presenting with EE will require initial emergent antiepileptic therapy (first-line drugs) and urgent controller therapy (second-line drugs) plus maintenance therapy, even if they are immediately controlled. By definition, in refractory EE, third and fourth line therapy is reserved for those who fail the previous two (27).

Intravenous (IV) administration is preferred; however, therapy can be administered intramuscularly (IM), rectally, intranasally (IN) or orally when IV is not possible. For IV therapy, lorazepam is the agent of choice; midazolam is preferred for IM therapy (it can also be administered nasally or orally) and diazepam for rectal (19).

The American Epilepsy Society guideline concluded that lorazepam and IV diazepam are equally effective in stopping seizures lasting at least five minutes. Likewise, rectal diazepam, IM, IN and oral midazolam are good at stopping seizures lasting at least five minutes. He concludes that there are three equivalent first-line options: lorazepam IV (0.1 mg/kg/dose; repeat if necessary), diazepam IV (0.15-0.2 mg/kg/dose; repeat if necessary) and midazolam IM (10 mg for > 40 kg; 5 mg for 13-40 kg; single dose) (28).

Oral midazolam administration can be achieved by dripping the appropriate dose between the cheek and gum with the patient in the recovery position. Absorption through this technique is better than swallowing. IN administration is achieved by instilling the appropriate dose in drops into the nostril (34).

The two most common intravenous benzodiazepines are lorazepam and diazepam. Diazepam has a high lipid solubility and therefore the ability to rapidly cross the blood-brain barrier; it is effective in jugulating seizures when administered at doses of 0.1-0.3 mg/kg intravenously. However, due to subsequent redistribution of the drug into adipose tissue, the duration of anticonvulsant effect may be < 20 minutes. Diazepam, lorazepam and midazolam all reach effective brain concentrations rapidly, although diazepam is slightly faster (34).

The pharmacokinetics of midazolam - whose elimination half-life is 90-150 minutes, versus lorazepam (12-24 hours) and diazepam (48 hours) - favour it. The half-life of midazolam may increase in certain subpopulations and during EE, and its metabolism by cytochrome P450 3A4 may make it more susceptible to drug-drug interactions than lorazepam, which is glucuronidated. In children, non-IV midazolam is more effective than diazepam (34).

Since intravenous lorazepam is not available in Mexico and midazolam administered by any route is superior to diazepam, its use as a first-line drug is the cornerstone in the treatment of EE (4).

Second-line drugs

There is as yet no evidence to determine the superiority of one drug over another, and their use will depend on the experience of each centre and the therapeutic limitations of each drug, although there are clinical trials already completed that attempt to clarify this question (5).

Phenytoin: second step for seizures that do not subside after two doses of benzodiazepines and in seizures that, despite having subsided, have been prolonged (higher risk of recurrence). Maximum effect after 15 minutes. Initial dose: 20 mg/kg IV, rate 1 mg/kg/min (maximum dose 1500 mg/day). Dilution in physiological saline, as it is not compatible with glucose solutions, as it would precipitate and form microcrystals (17).

Potential adverse effects: arrhythmias, increased QT interval and hypotension; it is therefore important to monitor the electrocardiogram and blood pressure during administration (these effects are particularly associated with rapid administration). Contraindicated in patients with hypotension or arrhythmias. May not be useful in non-convulsive EE and myoclonic seizures, and may even trigger generalised EE in these patients. Maintenance dose: 7 mg/kg/day IV given every 12 to 8 hours. Maximum: 1500 mg/day. Start 12 to 24 hours after the loading dose. Doses should be adjusted gradually according to plasma phenytoin concentrations (23).

Phenytoin is considered an RE D drug according to the Food and Drugs Administration (FDA) classification, so precautions must be taken in its preparation and administration. Recommendations for its preparation: open and handle the ampoule in biological safety cabinets (BSC) IIb or sterile isolators (SA) with double gloves, gown and mask. If it is not possible to prepare in a cabinet, use eye and respiratory protection. Recommendations for administration: wear double gloves and gown; use eye protection when there is a risk of splashing and respiratory protection if there is a possibility of inhalation (29).

Valproic acid (VPA): in addition to being indicated in benzodiazepine-refractory EE, it can also be effective in children with phenytoin-refractory EE. Its advantage is that it does not produce respiratory depression and has little haemodynamic impact. Because of its ability to produce hepatotoxicity, it is contraindicated in children under two years of age, polymedicated patients, and suspected metabolic and mitochondrial disease (12).

Side effects also include haematological disturbances (pancytopenia), hyperammonaemia or haemorrhagic pancreatitis. Status dose: 20 mg/kg IV to pass in 5-10 min (maximum dose 1,000 mg/day). It is considered first choice in primary generalised epilepsy, as phenytoin can aggravate these types of epilepsy, in myoclonic and non-convulsive EE, and is also effective in EE with absences, tonic-clonic and Lennox-Gastaut syndrome. Maintenance: 1-2 mg/kg/hour (23).

Levetiracetam (LVT): has a broad spectrum of action and a good pharmacokinetic profile, with a mechanism of action related to the synaptic vesicle protein SV2A, which is involved in the release of presynaptic neurotransmitters. In addition, it inhibits high-voltage-activated calcium channels and reverses inhibition of negative allosteric modulators of GABA and glycine (29).

It has no known drug interactions, low protein binding, no liver metabolism, renal excretion and very high oral bioavailability. The intravenous dose for EE would be a 30-60 mg/kg load. It is administered diluted in 100 ml (SF5%, G5%, lactated Ringer's) over 10-15 minutes, followed by maintenance of 25-30 mg/kg every 12 hours. The most accepted indications are: myoclonic EE (after benzodiazepines and valproic) which may be worsened by phenytoin, and non-convulsive EE (21).

Phenobarbital (PBP): its use is currently practically limited to neonates. It is considered a third-line treatment due to its significant side effects. It causes respiratory depression and arterial hypotension secondary to peripheral vasodilatation and myocardial depression, especially after previous doses of benzodiazepines (19).

Lacosamide: an amino acid that acts by optimising the slow inactivation of sodium channels, producing stabilisation of hyperexcitable neuronal membranes. There are optimistic data on the use of lacosamide in EE in children, but although there are studies carried out in the paediatric age group, there is still not enough evidence to propose its use (28).

Third-line medicines.

They are used in refractory status epilepticus (REE), i.e. persistence of seizures despite first- and second-line administration. The therapeutic approach aims to achieve seizure control (any clinical and electroencephalographic signs of epileptic activity), neuroprotection and avoidance of systemic complications (23).

 Coma induction is the most common treatment after failure of first- and second-line drugs. Unfortunately, there is insufficient evidence to guide clinical practice and the goal of induced coma (seizure termination, pattern, flare-suppression or complete suppression of EEG activity), duration and weaning parameters are unclear (19).

In addition to the induction of coma with anaesthetic agents, the use of adjuvant therapies such as immunomodulator, ketogenic diet, hypothermia, electroconvulsive therapy and vagal stimulation could be considered despite their low level of evidence (11).

Induction and maintenance of coma requires admission to a paediatric intensive care unit with cardiorespiratory monitoring that should be complemented by continuous electroencephalographic monitoring, in addition to respiratory or haemodynamic support as required by the patient (12).

It is better to achieve a flare-suppression pattern than to suppress electrical activity to avoid the side effects of arterial hypotension on the central nervous system. In general, it is recommended to maintain the induced coma for 24-48 hours after cessation of EE and to progressively reduce it until withdrawal in 12-24 hours, always maintaining the second-line antiepileptic drug used. The most commonly used drugs for coma induction are midazolam, thiopental and propofol. There are no randomised studies comparing them, although in most protocols the most common drug used to initiate this phase is midazolam (18).

Forecast

The prognosis of patients with EE varies according to age, cause and duration of EE. The mortality rate is around 3%17,18. It is related to the underlying disease (the main determinant of mortality), respiratory, cardiac or metabolic complications (23).

Patients with acute and remote symptomatic EE are more likely to die and more so if refractory. Mortality rates for febrile EE are much lower at around 0.2%. Neurological sequelae that may follow EE include secondary epilepsy, behavioural disorders, cognitive impairment or focal neurological deficits (28).

Data in relation to EE sequelae are difficult to interpret because they may be related to the underlying disorder rather than the EE. In addition, neurocognitive assessment is often not available and sequelae are not always reported in detail. Younger age, female gender and long duration of EE are associated with worse outcome. According to age, sequelae in children under one year occur in 29%, between 1 and 3 years in 11%, and in those older than 3 years in 6%19 (17).

7. Frame of Reference

Status epilepticus (SE) is the most common neurological emergency in children, with an incidence of approximately 20 events per 100,000 children/year in the developed world. This condition has significant morbidity and mortality when not appropriately treated.1 It is associated with a short-term mortality of 0-3% and a long-term mortality of 7% (4).

Mortality is estimated at less than 3% in children, but up to 30% in adults, so the goal of therapy is rapid termination of clinical or electrical seizure activity. The most commonly reported triggers are fever (in 36% of cases), medication changes (20%), unclear causes (9%), metabolic damage (8%), congenital malformations (7%), anoxic events (5%) and others, such as trauma, vascular, infection, tumours and drugs (18).

Benzodiazepines are the first-line treatment for SE because they can rapidly control seizures (see "Efficacy and pharmacokinetics of benzodiazepines" below). The three most commonly used benzodiazepines to treat SE are lorazepam, diazepam and midazolam (4).

The highest mortality groups are patients with anoxia or underlying pathologies and, to a lesser extent, those with epilepsy and low concentrations of antiepileptic drugs. Immediate control of EE and timely detection of the cause are essential, as they have a direct impact on morbidity and mortality. The neurological sequelae can be very diverse; however, cognitive sequelae predominate, because these patients are subjected to diffuse cerebral hypoxia by various mechanisms, so that we can also find motor, sensory, etc. sequelae (11).

The importance of having an EE protocol is that it will allow us to save time and avoid delays in treatment, prevent errors and improve patient care. In this pathology it is fundamental, as different studies have shown that early initiation of treatment with first-line drugs, generally benzodiazepines (BZD), favours the resolution of the crisis and improves the prognosis, while others relate the delay in the initiation of EE treatment with a worse prognosis and an increase in morbidity and mortality (19).

In the Hospital del Niño DIF Hidalgo, in 2016, a treatment algorithm was developed based on international and national research and treatment guidelines, however, it has not been fully implemented, so there is a need to know the results that this will have after its application in this institution to determine whether or not there is a positive impact on patient care, so the results of this research will allow decisions to be made to provide timely care or redesign the algorithm to correctly treat this pathology (7).

8. Material and Methods

8.1 Research design

Quantitative, observational and prospective study, which describes the therapeutic alliance of the doctors to the treatment algorithm of the paediatric patient in status epilepticus at the Hospital del Niño DIF Hidalgo.

8.2 Population

Patients with an admission diagnosis of status epilepticus, attended to at the Niño DIF Hospital in Hidalgo.

8.3 Sampling

A sample was not applied; a total of 24 files were part of the protocol, with a diagnosis of status epilepticus, attended at the Niño DIF Hospital in Hidalgo during the period from December 2020 to December 2021.

No formula will be applied to determine the sample size, as all electronic records of patients with a diagnosis of status epilepticus admitted to the Niño DIF Hospital in Hidalgo during the period from December 2020 to December 2021 will be entered.

No formula will be applied to determine the sample size, as all electronic records of patients with a diagnosis of status epilepticus admitted to the Niño DIF Hospital in Hidalgo during the period from December 2020 to December 2021 will be entered.

8.4 Time and space limits

Patients admitted to the emergency department in status epilepticus at the Niño DIF Hospital in Hidalgo during the period from December 2020 to December 2021.

8.5 Selection criteria

All electronic records of patients diagnosed on admission as status epilepticus admitted to the Emergency Department of the Hospital Niño DIF Hidalgo in the period from December 2020 to December 2021.

Inclusion criteria.

All electronic records of patients diagnosed on admission as status epilepticus admitted to the Emergency Department of the Hospital Niño DIF Hidalgo in the period from December 2020 to December 2021 who meet the following criteria according to the ILAE 2017:

- Generalised tonic-clonic seizures lasting 5 minutes or more.

- Two or more generalised tonic-clonic seizures without recovery of alertness within 30 minutes.

- Focal status epilepticus with loss of consciousness is a duration of 10 minutes or two or more without regaining consciousness within 60 minutes.

- Epileptic Syndrome of absence epileptic seizures with a duration of 10 to 15 minutes.

Exclusion criteria

- Electronic file with incomplete medical notes.
- Patient who decides on voluntary discharge or who has refused medical treatment.

Elimination criteria

- Electronic files that do not meet the selection and inclusion criteria.

8.6 Data collection instrument

1. Prior to carrying out the research protocol, the medical staff (seconded and residents) will be informed and their informed consent will be requested in writing (appendix 3). Subsequently, training will be provided on the diagnosis of status epilepticus as well as the application and correct use of the algorithm for the treatment of patients with status epilepticus at the Hospital del Niño DIF Hidalgo.

2. In the Emergency Department, the assigned doctors (who will be in charge) will be asked to ensure that all patients diagnosed with status epilepticus are treated according to the treatment algorithm for patients with status epilepticus of the Hospital Niño DIF Hidalgo, and together with the paediatric resident will make a complete and detailed medical note on the clinical condition and treatment.

3. The researcher will review the medical notes registered in Histoclin of the patients with a diagnosis of Status Epilepticus and collect the information requested in the format in Annex 2,

eliminating all those who do not meet the inclusion criteria or present exclusion criteria, respectively, as the case may be.

4. With the information obtained, a descriptive analysis of the therapeutic alliance of the treating physicians to the treatment algorithm for patients with status epilepticus in the Niño DIF Hospital will be carried out, as well as its evolution, with the aim of assessing its effectiveness and whether or not there is a need to make adjustments to it.

8.7 Data collection procedure.

-A descriptive analysis of the therapeutic alliance of the treating physicians to the treatment algorithm for patients with status epilepticus in the Niño DIF Hospital will be carried out, as well as the evolution of this.

-With regard to the statistical analysis of the number of patients seen, the classification of status epilepticus they present and the time in which the status epilepticus is successfully jugulated, the mean, median, standard deviation, minimum and maximum will be obtained.

-To determine the therapeutic alliance to the algorithm of treatment of the patient in status epilepticus at the Niño DIF Hospital, we will use a scale created by us that will classify the patient into 3 large groups, giving each one a score.

- 2: Adhere to the choice of drug, dose, route and time of administration.
- 1: They do not comply with one of the elements described in the previous item.
- 0: Failure to meet two or more of the elements described under good.

The data obtained will be used to obtain the frequency of each one of them (see Annex No. 2). The Excel programme will be used.

8.8 Ethical consideration.

Regulation of the General Health Law on research for health.

ARTICLE 17. Research risk is considered to be the probability that the research subject will suffer harm as an immediate or delayed consequence of the study. For the purposes of these Regulations, research is classified into the following categories:

I. Research without risk: These are studies that employ retrospective documentary research techniques and methods and those in which no intervention or intentional modification is carried out on the physiological, psychological and social variables of the individuals participating in the study, including: questionnaires, interviews, review of clinical records and others, in which no sensitive aspects of their behaviour are identified or dealt with.

II. Minimal risk research: Prospective studies that employ data risk through procedures common to routine diagnostic or treatment physical or psychological examinations, including: subject weighing, hearing acuity tests; electrocardiogram, thermography, collection of excreta and external secretions, collection of placenta during delivery, collection of amniotic fluid at rupture of membranes, collection of saliva, decidual teeth and permanent teeth extracted for therapeutic indication, dental plaque and calculus removed by non-invasive prophylactic procedure, hair and nail clipping without causing disfigurement, blood collection by venipuncture in healthy adults, with a maximum frequency of twice a week and a maximum volume of 450 ml in two months, except during pregnancy, moderate exercise in healthy volunteers, psychological testing of individuals or groups in which the subject's behaviour will not be manipulated, research with commonly used medicines with a wide therapeutic margin, authorised for sale, using the established indications, doses and routes of administration and which are not investigational medicinal products as defined in Article 65 of this Regulation.

III.- Research with greater than minimal risk: These are those in which the probabilities of affecting the subject are significant, including: radiological and microwave studies, trials with the medicines and modalities defined in article 65 of these Regulations, trials with new devices, studies that include surgical procedures, blood extraction of more than 2% of the circulating volume in neonates, amniocentesis and other invasive techniques or major procedures, those that employ randomised methods of assignment to therapeutic schemes and those that have placebo control, among others.

For the purposes of these Regulations, pharmacological research is understood to be the scientific activities aimed at the study of medicines and biological products for human use, for which there is no previous experience in the country, which have not been registered by the Secretariat and, therefore, are not commercially distributed, as well as medicines registered and approved (sic DOF 06-01-1987) for sale, when their use is investigated with modalities, indications, doses or routes of administration different from those established, including their use in combinations.

According to article 65 of the Regulations of the General Health Law on Health Research, our protocol does not qualify as pharmacological research because we will be using drugs already approved by the Ministry of Health. Due to the provisions of article 17 of this law, we would classify it as research with minimal risk, as we use a treatment algorithm based on drugs, route, dose and duration of infusion already established in both international and national guidelines (see Annexes 1 and 3).

9. Results

9.1 Socio-demographic data

Graph No.1 Sex of patients

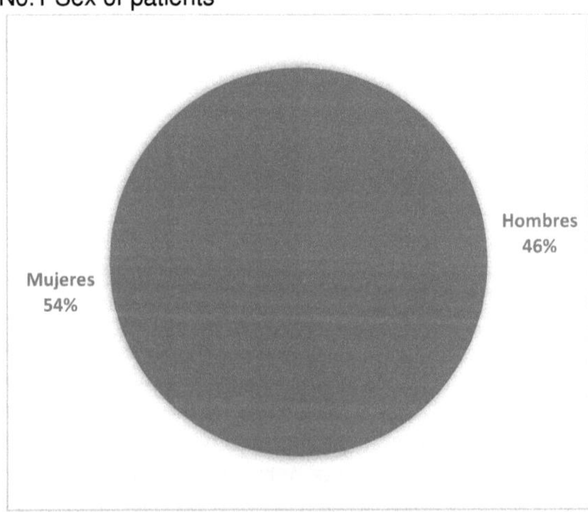

Source: N=24 Histoclin 2020-2021-Hospital del Niño DIF

In the DIF Hidalgo Children's Hospital, a total of 24 patients were attended from December 2020 to December 2021 (13 female cases

(54.1%) and 11 male cases (45.9%)), with an average of 2 patients per month.

Graph No.2 Age of patients

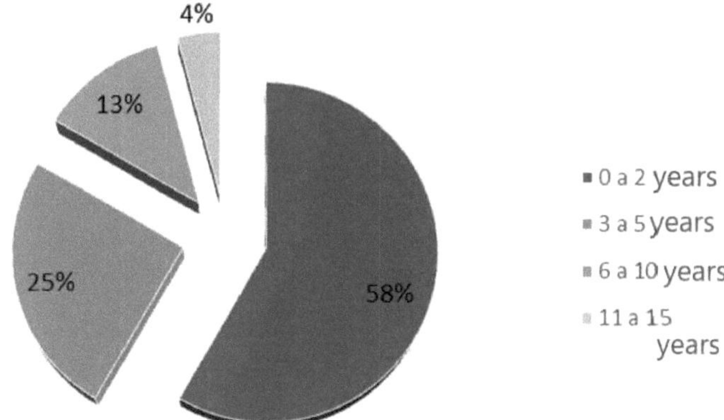

Source: N=24. Histoclin 2020-2021-Hospital del Niño DIF.

9.2 Instrument data

With the following age ranges 0 months to 2 years (14), 3 to 5 years (6), 6 to 10 years (3) and 11 to 15 years (1). With an average age of 36 months.

Graph No.3 Classification of status epilepticus

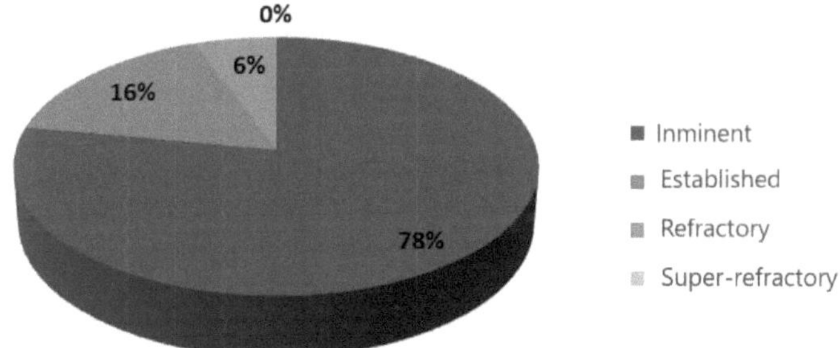

Source: N=24. Histoclin 2020-2021-Hospital del Niño DIF.

These were classified as impending status epilepticus, 19 cases (77.9%), 4 established (16.4%), 3 refractory (5.7%) and no super-refractory cases.

Graph No.4 Therapeutic alliance to the treatment algorithm for patients with status epilepticus in the Hospital del Niño DIF Hidalgo.

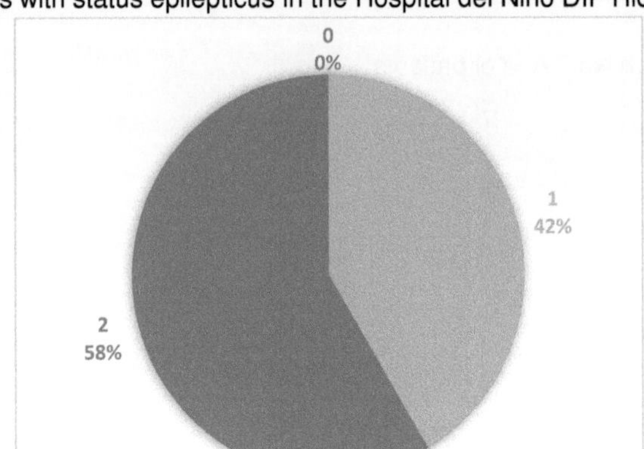

Source: N=24. Histoclin 2020-2021-Hospital del Niño DIF.

2: Adhere to the choice of drug, dose, route and time of administration.
1: They do not comply with one of the elements described in the previous item.
0: Failure to meet two or more of the elements described under good.

The therapeutic alliance to the treatment algorithm for patients with status epilepticus, 58.33% of the physicians adhere to the choice of drug, dosage, route and time of administration, while 41.67% fail in one of these elements, mainly the drug dosage.

With respect to the time in which the patient was jugulated, status epilepticus lasted an average of 29.8 minutes, with a mean of 20 minutes and a mode of 15 minutes, with a minimum of 5 minutes and a maximum of 120 minutes, thus generating a standard deviation of± 26.6 minutes. The average length of stay in hospital for these patients was 1.2 days, with a minimum of 1 day and a maximum of 4 days. It should be noted that those who were hospitalised for the longest time were not due to status epilepticus but to their underlying disease or because most of them had an infectious condition that required days of intravenous antibiotics.

Comparing the results of this research with those obtained in the 2018 preview, we obtain the following information.

Description	2021	2016
Duration of the EE	DE 26.6	DE 33.8

Cerebral ischaemia	0%	13.7%
Sepsis	0%	6.8%
Death	No cases were submitted	Mortality rate of 0.6 per 1000 patients.
Main aetiology	Infectious	Infectious

Table 7: Comparison between the results obtained from the 2016 research compared to 2021.

10. Discussion

After the implementation of the algorithm for patients with status epilepticus at the Hospital del Niño DIF, no study had been carried out to demonstrate its efficacy in our institution, so this study made it possible to ascertain the doctors' adherence to it.

During the study protocol period from December 2021 to 2022, more women than men were attended with a ratio (M : F) of 1.18:1, although this is not as significant a change from the results obtained in a previous study in our hospital in 2018, where more men than women were attended (F : F) 1.2:1 (7).

100% of the cases registered as status epilepticus were classified appropriately, the type of status epilepticus continues to prevail the imminent, with 77.9% of cases, the time in jugular status epilepticus decreased by 4 minutes, previously with a DE 33.9 minutes and now of 26.6 minutes, which was the result of a better therapeutic alliance to the treatment algorithm because 58.33% of the physicians did it properly in terms of choice of drug, dose, route and time of administration, while 41.67% failed in one of these elements, mainly in the dose of the drug.

Although most international guidelines, as well as the Algorithm of the Hospital del Niño, DIF, consider diazepam to be the drug of choice for treating status epilepticus, due to the pandemic we are currently experiencing as a result of COVID 2019, this benzodiazepine was in short supply, so midazolam was used more as the first-line drug. The choice of medication coincides with the different articles on which our research is based, where benzodiazepines are considered to be the group of choice as first-line drugs to treat status epilepticus (4).

The doctors at Niño DIF had an adequate choice of medication for the treatment of patient EE according to our algorithm, failing in the dosage of medication, because some used a lower or higher dosage than recommended.

A comparison with previous research data from our hospital shows that there has been a significant improvement in the care of patients with status epilepticus in our institution, with a reduction in the duration of the condition and the number of days of hospital stay, as well as no morbidity such as sepsis, cerebral ischaemia or death. The patients with longer hospital stays were not due to status epilepticus, but because some of them required intravenous antibiotics for the infection they presented.   Therefore, we can conclude that a treatment algorithm improves patient prognosis by reducing morbidity and mortality and the number of days of in-hospital stay (11).

When using fourth-line drugs for the treatment of status epilepticus, we must consider that the patient already has neuronal damage due to the duration of the event, which is estimated to be longer than 30 minutes, increasing the possibility of brain death secondary to hypoxia; the risk of this complication is greater when Thiopental is used, as it generates cerebral ischaemia as an adverse effect. During the year of our protocol, there were no cases of brain death, and by adhering adequately to the algorithm, control of status epilepticus was achieved with first and second line drugs.

Following the data obtained, we consider it necessary to have equipment in the Emergency Department to be able to perform an electroencephalogram on all patients with status epilepticus who arrive at our Unit, to corroborate that they were referred both clinically and electrically, in order to avoid misdiagnosis, considering that because they do not present movements the condition has subsided and that they may still be electrically active, which represents a risk factor for brain damage and affects the quality of life of the patients.

11. Conclusions and recommendations

Conclusion

The present study shows that having an algorithm for the treatment of ES, as well as the complete therapeutic alliance to it, improves the prognosis of our patients by reducing morbidity and mortality.

It is essential to have medicines readily available for patient care in the emergency department, so it would be appropriate to have a trolley in the emergency room that contains what is needed for treatment.

Electroencephalographic monitoring is necessary for all patients with EE, on all shifts, in order to corroborate the cessation of electrical activity, as rapid identification and proper management of EE is an important prognostic factor in preventing neurological and/or systemic complications.

Recommendations

Continue with the ongoing training and use of the algorithm for patients with status epilepticus at the Hospital del Niño DIF, Hidalgo.

A trolley containing the medicines necessary for the treatment of patients with status epilepticus should be kept in the Emergency Department of our unit in order to ensure that these medicines are available to provide adequate and timely treatment to our patients.

We must have an electroencephalogram on all shifts in order to be able to monitor brain electrical activity to corroborate the end of status epilepticus both clinically and electrically.

Bibliography

1. Ngugi A.K, Kariuki SM, Bottomley C, Kleinschmidt I, Sander JW Newton CR. Incidence of epilepsy. Neurology. 2011; 77: 1005-1012.
2. Kirsten M, Khara M. Samuel MD, Scott B. Patten MD, Churl-Su K, Jonathan D. Prevalence and incidence of epilepsy A systematic review and meta-analysis of international studies. Neurology. 2017; 88: 296-303.
3. Scheffer IE, Berkovic S, Capovilla G, Connolly Mb, French J, Hirsch E, et al. ILAE classification of epilepsies. Epilepsia. 2017; 58(4):512-521.
4. Reséndiz-Aparicio JC. Clinical guidelines of the Priority Epilepsy Program of the Health Sector, Mexico. Rev Mex Neurosci. 2019; 20(3):56-128.
5. Oliva-Meza HOM Ochoa-Morales X. Neural party: status epilepticus in paediatrics. An Med (Mex). 2018; 63 (1): 38-47.
6. Douglas M. Smith, Emily J. McGinnis, Diana J. Management of Status Epilepticus in Children. J. Clin. Med. 2016; 47(5): 1-19.
7. Lopez-Alamilla AA. Evaluation of the management of status epilepticus in the Hospital del Niño DIF from 2011 to 2016. [Specialty thesis] . Mexico: UAEH; 2018 : http://dgsa.uaeh.edu.mx:8080/bibliotecadigital/handle/231104/224 2
8. Gretchen MB, Rodney B, Jan C, Brian A, Thomas PB. Guidelines for the Evaluation and Management of Status Epilepticus. Neurocrit Care. 2012; 56 (3): 567-578.
9. Bello N, Calvo-Medina R, Mora-Ramírez MD, Ramos-Fernández JM.Status epilepticus in paediatric patients: evolutionary consequences and epidemiological update. Rev Neurol 2020;71 (10):365-372.
10. Fallahian F, Hashemian SM. Critical Management of Status Epilepticus. J Clin Intensive Care Med. 2017; 2: 001-015.
11. JN Friedman. Emergency management of thepaediatric patient with generalized convulsivestatus epilepticus. Paediatr Child Health 2011;16(2):91-7.
12. Eugen T, Hannah C, Dale H, Andrea OR, Scheffer I, Shlomo S, Simon S, Lowenstein SI. A definition and classification of status epilepticus - Report of the ILAE Task Force on Classification of Status Epilepticus. Epilepsia. 2015; 56(10):1515-1523.
13. Moreno-Medinilla EE, Negrillo-Ruano R, Calvo-Medina R, Mora-Ramírez MD, Martínez-Antón JL. Status epilepticus in paediatrics:

retrospective study and review of the literature.Rev Neurol. 2015 May 1;60(9):394-400.

14. Malagón- Valdez J. Status epilepticus in childhood. Medicina (B Aires). 2013;73 Suppl 1:77-82.

15. Paz-Vargas C, Varela X, Kleinsteuber K, Cortés R, Avaria MA. Review of paediatric convulsive status epilepticus and its antiepileptic management. Rev Med Chile .2016; 144: 83-93.

16. Vaccarezza M, Silva W, Maxit C, Agosta G. Super-refractory status epilepticus: treatment with ketogenic diet in pediatrics. Rev Neurol. 2012 Jul 1;55(1):20-5. Spanish. PMID: 22718405.

17. Cardoso I, Acevedo K, Hernández M, Santin J, Moya P, Godoy J, Castillo A, Soto P, Mesa T. Refractory status epilepticus in children: characterisation of epilepsies, continuous electroencephalographic monitoring and response to treatment. Rev Neurol. 2013. 16;56(8):401-8.

18. Trinka E, Cock H, Hesdorffer D, Rossetti A. Adefinition and classification of status epilepticus. Report of the ILAE Task Force on Classification of Status Epilepticus. Epilepsia.2015:56(10):1515-1523.

19. Abend NS, Bearden D, Helbig I, Mc-Guire J. Status epilepticus and refactory status epilepticus management. Semin Pediatr Neurol. 2014; 21(4):263-274.

20. Kurz JE, Goldstein J. Status Epilepticus in the Pediatric Emergency Department. Clin Pediatr Emerg Med. 2015 Mar 1;16(1):37-47.

21. McKenzie KC, Hahn CD, Friedman JN. Emergency management of the paediatric patient with convulsive status epilepticus. Paediatr Child Health 2021; 26:50-78.

22. Brophy GM, Bell R, Claassen J, et al. Guidelines for the evaluation and management of status epilepticus. Neurocrit Care. 2012; 17:3-23.

23. Gaínza-Lein M, Sánchez Fernández I, Jackson M, et al. Association of Time to Treatment With Short-term Outcomes for Pediatric Patients With Refractory Convulsive Status Epilepticus. JAMA Neurol. 2018; 75:410-425.

24. Sánchez Fernández I, Abend NS, Agadi S, et al. Time from convulsive status epilepticus onset to anticonvulsant administration in children. Neurology. 2015; 84:2304-2345.

25. Chin RF, Neville BG, Peckham C, et al. Treatment of community-onset, childhood convulsive status epilepticus: a prospective, population-based study. Lancet Neurol .2008; 7:696-689.

26. McTague A, Martland T, Appleton R. Drug management for acute tonic-clonic seizures including convulsive status epilepticus in children. Cochrane Database Syst Rev. 2018; 1: 195-208.

27. Chamberlain JM, Okada P, Holsti M, et al. Lorazepam vs diazepam for pediatric status epilepticus: a randomized clinical trial. JAMA.2014; 311:1652-1678.

28. Vasquez A, Gaínza-Lein M, Abend NS, et al. First-line medication dosing in pediatric refractory status epilepticus. Neurology.2020; 95:26-83.

29. Chin RF, Verhulst L, Neville BG, et al. Inappropriate emergency management of status epilepticus in children contributes to need for intensive care. J Neurol Neurosurg Psychiatry .2004; 75:158-1674.

30. Alshehri A, Abulaban A, Bokhari R, et al. Intravenous Versus Nonintravenous Benzodiazepines for the Cessation of Seizures: A Systematic Review and Meta-analysis of Randomized Controlled Trials. Acad Emerg Med. 2017; 24:875-890.

31. Reig Sáenz R, Sánchez Mirallesb A,Herrera Murilloa M, González Lorenzoa M, Martínez Salcedocy E , Almanza-Lopez S. Poor prognostic factors in convulsive status epilepticus. An Pediatr (Barc).2005;63(4):307-313.

32. Qureshi A, Wassmer E, Davies P, et al. Comparative audit of intravenous lorazepam and diazepam in the emergency treatment of convulsive status epilepticus in children. Seizure. 2002; 11:141-1150.

33. Ahmad S, Ellis JC, Kamwendo H, Molyneux E. Efficacy and safety of intranasal lorazepam versus intramuscular paraldehyde for protracted seizures in children: an open randomised trial. Lancet. 2006; 367:1591-1598.

34. McIntyre J, Robertson S, Norris E. Safety and efficacy of buccal midazolam versus rectal diazepam for emergency treatment of seizures in children: a randomised controlled trial. Lancet. 2005; 366:205-215.

35. Alansari K, Barkat M, Mohamed AH. Intramuscular Versus Buccal Midazolam for Pediatric Seizures: A Randomized Double-Blinded Trial. Pediatr Neurol.2020; 109:28-39.

36. Silbergleit R, Durkalski V, Lowenstein D. Intramuscular versus intravenous therapy for prehospital status epilepticus. N Engl J Med .2012; 366:591-597.

37. Welch RD, Nicholas K, Durkalski-Mauldin VL, et al. Intramuscular midazolam versus intravenous lorazepam for the prehospital

treatment of status epilepticus in the pediatric population. Epilepsia. 2015; 56:254-276.

Annex. No. 1 Office of the Ethics Committee

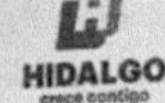

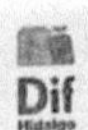

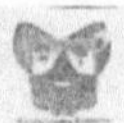

HNDH-CEI. Of. No. 141/02/2021

M.C. Salvador Jiménez Mejines
Médico Residente de segundo año
Presente

Pachuca, de Soto Hgo., a 02 de febrero del 2021.

Número de registro de protocolo de Investigación

Por este medio le informo que se ha revisado su protocolo de investigación bajo los preceptos establecidos por la Ley General de Salud en materia de Investigación en Salud y la NOM-012-SSA3-2012, que establece los criterios para la ejecución de proyectos de investigación para la salud en seres humanos. Por tanto, se aprueba la ejecución del proyecto de investigación con número de solicitud CICEICB-2020-37-03 y titulado: **"Adherencia al algoritmo de tratamiento del paciente pediátrico en estado epiléptico del Hospital del Niño DIF Hidalgo."**, otorgando el número de registro:

CICEICB-EP2021-11

Se le solicita que, a partir de la fecha, indique este número en todos los documentos de difusión científica derivados de esta investigación y al finalizar su proyecto, deberá notificar vía oficio la terminación del mismo a los Comités de Investigación del Hospital del Niño DIF Hidalgo. Finalmente, se le invita que realice las actividades de Investigación en el Hospital de acuerdo a las Buenas Prácticas Clínicas y a los preceptos de ética, metodología científica y bioseguridad, apegados a la normatividad.

Este documento tiene vigencia hasta el 30 de noviembre de 2021.

Atentamente

Dra. Mónica Langarica Bulos
Directora del hospital del Niño DIF
Presidenta del Comité de Investigación
y del Comité de Bioseguridad

Dr. Felipe Arteaga García
Coordinador de Enseñanza e Inv.
Presidente del Comité de Ética en Inv.

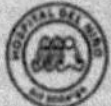

Annex No. 2 Operationalisation of variables.

VARIABLE	DESCRIPTION	TYPE	UNIT OF MEASUREMENT OR CLASSIFICATION
Status epilepticus	Seizure lasting more than 5 minutes without recovery.	Discrete quantitative	Yes/No
Classification of status epilepticus	It is determined from the duration of status epilepticus on admission to the Emergency Department.	Discrete quantitative	0= Incipient (5 -30 minutes) 1= Established (30-60 minutes) 2= Refractory (1 hour to 24 hours) 3=Superrefractory (More than 24 hours)

	Amount of medicine administered during a specified period of time -Diazepam Rectal: 0.5 mgkgdo Intravenous: 0.3-05mgkgdo -Phenytoin sodium 20mgkgdo -Phenytoin sodium supplement 10mgkgdo -Levetiracetam 30-60mgkg -Midazola 2mgkghora -Thiopental 2-7mgkghora. -Propofol 30-250 mcgkgmin -Ketamine 0.63-7.5mgkghora	Discrete quantitative	Yes/No
Administrati on of drug doses			
Route of administrati on	The means by which the medicinal product is administered. -Diazepam: intrarectal or intravenous. Phenytoin, valproic acid, levetiracetam, midazolam, thiopental, propofol, ketamine: intravenous.	Discrete quantitative	Yes/No
Infusion time	The duration of intravenous administration of drugs and fluids. DFH 1 mlkgminute Thiopental:1-5 mg/kg/h.	Discrete quantitative	Yes/No

Therapeutic alliance to the algorithm	Action to follow an established therapeutic plan	Discrete quantitative	-2: Adhere to the choice of drug, dose, route and time of administration. -1: They do not comply with one of the elements described in the previous item. -0: Do not adhere to two or more of the elements described in good.
Jugular status epilepticus	Time elapsed from initiation of first-line treatment to the cessation of status epilepticus	Discrete quantitative	Minutes

Annex No. 3 Informed Consent.

It will be used electronically and will be filled out in Histoclin.

INFORMED CONSENT

Pachuca, Hidalgo, Hidalgo, on the

I ____declare that I have been informed and invited to participate in an investigation entitled: **"THERAPEUTIC ALLIANCE OF THE PHYSICIANS TO THE TREATMENT ALGORITHM OF THE PEDIATRIC PATIENT IN EPILEPTIC STATE, OF THE HOSPITAL DEL NIÑO DIF HIDALGO"**, this is a scientific research project that has the support of the Hospital del Niño DIF, Hidalgo. I understand that this study seeks to know: the therapeutic alliance of the Doctors to the algorithm of treatment of the paediatric patient in status epilepticus of the Hospital del Niño DIF Hidalgo, and I know that my participation will be carried out in the Hospital del Niño DIF, Hidalgo. It has been explained to me that the information registered will be confidential, and that the names of the participants will be associated with a serial number, this means that the results will not be known by other people nor will they be identified in the phase of publication of the results. I am aware that the data will not be given to me and that there will be no remuneration for participation in this study, but that this information may benefit indirectly and therefore has a societal benefit given the research being conducted. I also know that I can refuse to participate or withdraw at any stage of the research, without expression of cause or negative consequences to me. Yes. I voluntarily agree to participate in this study and have received a copy of this document.

If you have any questions during any stage of the study, please contact Salvador Jiménez Mejines, Third Grade Resident at the Hospital del Niño, DIF Hidalgo.

Participant's signature.
Witness

Printed by Books on Demand GmbH, Norderstedt / Germany